Table of Contents

INTRODUCTION

A low blood sugar diet, also known as a hypoglycemia diet, is a dietary approach that aims to manage the symptoms of low blood sugar (hypoglycemia). Hypoglycemia occurs when blood sugar levels drop below normal levels, usually below 70 milligrams per deciliter (mg/dL). Symptoms can vary but may include dizziness, confusion, shakiness, and fatigue. A low blood sugar diet involves eating small, frequent meals throughout the day to help stabilize blood sugar levels. This typically involves balancing macronutrients, such as eating lean proteins, whole grains, and vegetables while avoiding refined carbohydrates and added sugars. The goal is to maintain a steady stream of glucose in the bloodstream to prevent blood sugar spikes and crashes. A low blood sugar diet may be recommended for people who experience hypoglycemia due to diabetes, reactive hypoglycemia, or other medical conditions. It is important to work with a healthcare provider or registered dietitian to develop an individualized plan that meets nutritional needs and manages hypoglycemia symptoms. In addition to dietary changes, lifestyle factors such as regular exercise, stress management, and adequate sleep may also play a role in managing hypoglycemia.

Explanation of low blood sugar (hypoglycemia) and its causes

Low blood sugar, also known as hypoglycemia, is a condition that occurs when the level of glucose (sugar) in the blood drops below the normal range. In most people, a blood glucose level of less than 70 mg/dL is considered hypoglycemia. Glucose is the primary source of energy for the body's cells, including the brain. Normally, the body maintains a stable blood sugar level through a complex system of hormones and enzymes that regulate the release of glucose from the liver and the uptake of glucose by the cells. However, certain factors can disrupt this balance and lead to hypoglycemia. The most common causes of hypoglycemia include:

1. Diabetes: People with diabetes may experience hypoglycemia if they take too much insulin or other diabetes medications, skip meals, or exercise more than usual.

2. Reactive hypoglycemia: Some people may experience hypoglycemia a few hours after eating a meal that is high in sugar or refined carbohydrates.

3. Alcohol consumption: Drinking alcohol can cause hypoglycemia by interfering with the liver's ability to release glucose into the bloodstream.

4. Other medical conditions: Certain medical conditions such as liver disease, kidney disease, and pancreatic tumors can cause hypoglycemia.

Symptoms of hypoglycemia can vary but may include shakiness, sweating, confusion, dizziness, and fatigue. In severe cases, hypoglycemia can lead to seizures or loss of consciousness. It is important to work with a healthcare provider to identify the underlying cause of hypoglycemia and develop a treatment plan.

Overview of how a low blood sugar diet can help manage hypoglycemia

A low blood sugar diet is a dietary approach that can help manage hypoglycemia by regulating the release of glucose into the bloodstream. By consuming small, frequent meals throughout the day that are balanced in macronutrients, people with hypoglycemia can help prevent blood sugar spikes and crashes.

When the body receives a sudden influx of sugar, such as from a high-carbohydrate meal, the pancreas releases insulin to help move glucose out of the bloodstream and into the cells. However, if too much insulin is released, or if glucose is used up quickly, blood sugar levels can drop rapidly, leading to hypoglycemia. A low blood sugar diet can help prevent this by encouraging the consumption of complex carbohydrates, such as whole grains, fruits, and vegetables, which are broken down more slowly and provide a more sustained release of glucose into the bloodstream. Eating protein with meals can also help slow the absorption of carbohydrates and further stabilize blood sugar levels. In addition to balancing macronutrients, a low blood sugar diet may also involve limiting or avoiding foods that can cause blood sugar spikes, such as refined carbohydrates and sugary drinks. People with hypoglycemia may also benefit from eating a small, high-protein snack before bed to help prevent overnight hypoglycemia. Overall, a low blood sugar diet can be an effective way to manage hypoglycemia symptoms and prevent dangerous drops in blood sugar levels. It is important to work with a healthcare provider or registered dietitian to develop an individualized plan that meets nutritional needs and manages hypoglycemia symptoms.

Principles of a Low Blood Sugar Diet

The principles of a low blood sugar diet involve balancing macronutrients and eating small, frequent meals throughout the day to help stabilize blood sugar levels. Here are some key principles of a low blood sugar diet:

1. Eat small, frequent meals: Eating small, frequent meals throughout the day, rather than three large meals, can help keep blood sugar levels stable. Aim for 5-6 meals per day, spaced out every 2-3 hours.

2. Balance macronutrients: Balancing macronutrients, such as carbohydrates,

proteins, and fats, can help prevent blood sugar spikes and crashes. A balanced meal should contain lean protein, complex carbohydrates, and healthy fats.

3. Emphasize complex carbohydrates: Complex carbohydrates, such as whole grains, fruits, and vegetables, are broken down more slowly and provide a more sustained release of glucose into the bloodstream.

4. Avoid or limit refined carbohydrates and added sugars: Refined carbohydrates, such as white bread and pasta, and sugary drinks can cause blood sugar spikes and crashes. Limit or avoid these foods as much as possible.

5. Include lean protein: Protein can help slow the absorption of carbohydrates and further stabilize blood sugar levels. Lean protein sources include chicken, fish, tofu, and legumes.

6. Choose healthy fats: Healthy fats, such as those found in nuts, seeds, avocado, and olive oil, can help slow the absorption of carbohydrates and provide a feeling of satiety.

7. Avoid alcohol: Drinking alcohol can cause hypoglycemia by interfering with the liver's ability to release glucose into the bloodstream.

Overall, the principles of a low blood sugar diet involve eating a balanced, nutrient-dense diet that emphasizes complex carbohydrates, lean protein, and healthy fats while avoiding or limiting refined carbohydrates and added sugars. It is important to work with a healthcare provider or registered dietitian to develop an individualized plan that meets nutritional needs and manages hypoglycemia symptoms.

Explanation of the main principles of a low blood sugar diet, such as eating small, frequent meals

The main principles of a low blood sugar diet are designed to help regulate blood sugar levels by balancing macronutrients and eating small, frequent meals throughout the day. Here is a more detailed explanation of some of the main principles:

1. Eating small, frequent meals: Consuming small, frequent meals throughout the day can help maintain steady blood sugar levels. This is because smaller meals are easier for the body to process and require less insulin to transport glucose into the cells. Eating every 2-3 hours can help prevent blood sugar spikes and crashes that can occur with larger, less frequent meals.

2. Balancing macronutrients: Balancing macronutrients, such as carbohydrates, protein, and fats, is essential for maintaining stable blood sugar levels. Complex carbohydrates, such as whole grains, fruits, and vegetables, provide a steady source of glucose for the body, while lean protein and healthy fats help slow the absorption of carbohydrates, preventing blood sugar spikes and crashes.

3. Emphasizing complex carbohydrates: Complex carbohydrates are important for a low blood sugar diet because they are broken down more slowly and provide a more sustained release of glucose into the bloodstream. Examples of complex carbohydrates include whole grains, fruits, and vegetables.

4. Limiting refined carbohydrates and added sugars: Refined carbohydrates and

added sugars can cause rapid spikes in blood sugar levels, followed by crashes. Foods to limit or avoid on a low blood sugar diet include white bread, pasta, sugary drinks, candy, and other sweets.

5. Including lean protein: Lean protein is an essential component of a low blood sugar diet because it helps slow the absorption of carbohydrates and provides a feeling of satiety. Examples of lean protein sources include chicken, fish, tofu, and legumes.

6. Choosing healthy fats: Healthy fats, such as those found in nuts, seeds, avocado, and olive oil, can help slow the absorption of carbohydrates and provide a feeling of satiety. Including healthy fats in meals and snacks can also help prevent hunger and overeating.

Overall, the main principles of a low blood sugar diet are designed to promote balanced eating habits that support stable blood sugar levels throughout the day. It is important to work with a healthcare provider or registered dietitian to develop an individualized plan that meets nutritional needs and manages hypoglycemia symptoms.

Importance of balancing macronutrients and avoiding refined carbohydrates and added sugars

Balancing macronutrients and avoiding refined carbohydrates and added sugars are both crucial components of a low blood sugar diet for managing hypoglycemia. Here's why:

Balancing macronutrients: Macronutrients are the main nutrients that make up our diet, including carbohydrates, protein, and fat. A diet that is high in carbohydrates and low in protein and fat can cause blood sugar spikes and crashes, as the body will need to produce more insulin to process the excess glucose from the carbohydrates. Eating a balanced diet that includes a combination of complex carbohydrates, lean protein, and healthy fats can help prevent these blood sugar fluctuations and stabilize blood sugar levels. Avoiding refined carbohydrates and added sugars: Refined carbohydrates, such as white bread, pasta, and sugary drinks, are quickly broken down into glucose and absorbed into the bloodstream, causing rapid spikes in blood sugar levels. Similarly, added sugars found in candy, baked goods, and other sweets can cause blood sugar spikes and crashes. Over time, consuming too many refined carbohydrates and added sugars can lead to insulin resistance, a condition in which the body becomes less responsive to insulin and is unable to regulate blood sugar levels effectively. By avoiding or limiting refined carbohydrates and added sugars, individuals with hypoglycemia can help prevent blood sugar fluctuations and promote stable blood sugar levels throughout the day. Instead, they should focus on consuming complex carbohydrates, lean protein, and healthy fats to provide a steady source of energy and prevent hunger and overeating. Working with a healthcare provider or registered dietitian can help individuals develop a personalized low blood sugar diet plan that meets their nutritional needs and supports stable blood sugar levels.

Foods to Eat on a Low Blood Sugar Diet

When following a low blood sugar diet, it is important to choose foods that help stabilize blood sugar levels and provide sustained energy throughout the day. Here are some examples of foods to eat on a low blood sugar diet:

1. Complex carbohydrates: Examples of complex carbohydrates include whole grains (such as brown rice, quinoa, and whole wheat bread), fruits (such as berries, apples, and citrus fruits), and vegetables (such as leafy greens, broccoli, and carrots).

2. Lean protein: Examples of lean protein sources include chicken, turkey, fish, tofu, tempeh, legumes (such as lentils and beans), and low-fat dairy products (such as yogurt and cottage cheese).

3. Healthy fats: Examples of healthy fats include nuts and seeds (such as almonds, walnuts, chia seeds, and flaxseeds), avocado, olive oil, and fatty fish (such as salmon and tuna).

4. Non-starchy vegetables: Non-starchy vegetables are low in carbohydrates and calories and high in fiber, making them a great choice for a low blood sugar diet. Examples include leafy greens, broccoli, cauliflower, cucumber, tomatoes, and bell peppers.

5. Low-sugar fruits: While fruits are a great source of vitamins and minerals, some are higher in sugar than others. Low-sugar fruit options include berries, citrus fruits, apples, and pears.

6. Water: Drinking plenty of water throughout the day is important for staying hydrated and promoting healthy blood sugar levels.

By focusing on whole, unprocessed foods that are high in fiber, protein, and healthy fats, individuals with hypoglycemia can help prevent blood sugar spikes and crashes and promote stable blood sugar levels. It is important to work with a healthcare provider or registered dietitian to develop a personalized low blood sugar diet plan that meets individual nutritional needs and supports stable blood sugar levels.

Overview of foods that are good to eat on a low blood sugar diet, such as lean proteins, whole grains, and vegetables

A low blood sugar diet emphasizes whole, unprocessed foods that are rich in nutrients and fiber, and that help stabilize blood sugar levels. Here's an overview of some of the foods that are good to eat on a low blood sugar diet:

1. Lean proteins: Lean proteins, such as chicken, turkey, fish, tofu, tempeh, legumes (such as lentils and beans), and low-fat dairy products (such as yogurt and cottage cheese), provide the body with sustained energy and help prevent blood sugar crashes.

2. Whole grains: Whole grains, such as brown rice, quinoa, whole wheat bread, and oatmeal, are high in fiber and complex carbohydrates, which help slow down the absorption of glucose into the bloodstream and promote stable blood sugar levels.

3. Non-starchy vegetables: Non-starchy vegetables, such as leafy greens, broccoli, cauliflower, cucumber, tomatoes, and bell peppers, are low in calories and carbohydrates and high in fiber, which

helps promote satiety and stable blood sugar levels.

4. Low-sugar fruits: Low-sugar fruits, such as berries, citrus fruits, apples, and pears, are high in fiber, vitamins, and minerals and can provide a healthy source of carbohydrates without causing blood sugar spikes.

5. Healthy fats: Healthy fats, such as nuts and seeds (such as almonds, walnuts, chia seeds, and flaxseeds), avocado, olive oil, and fatty fish (such as salmon and tuna), provide the body with a steady source of energy and help keep blood sugar levels stable.

By incorporating these foods into a low blood sugar diet and avoiding or limiting refined carbohydrates and added sugars, individuals with hypoglycemia can help prevent blood sugar spikes and crashes and promote stable blood sugar levels throughout the day. It is important to work with a healthcare provider or registered dietitian to develop a personalized low blood sugar diet plan that meets individual nutritional needs and supports stable blood sugar levels.

Foods to Avoid on a Low Blood Sugar Diet

When following a low blood sugar diet, it is important to avoid or limit certain foods that can cause blood sugar spikes and crashes. Here are some examples of foods to avoid on a low blood sugar diet:

1. Refined carbohydrates: Foods made with refined carbohydrates, such as white bread, pasta, and pastries, can cause blood sugar levels to spike quickly and then crash shortly thereafter.

2. Sugary drinks: Sugary drinks, such as soda, fruit juice, and sports drinks, are

high in added sugars and can cause blood sugar spikes.

3. Processed and packaged snacks: Many processed and packaged snacks, such as chips, crackers, and cookies, are high in refined carbohydrates and added sugars, which can cause blood sugar spikes and crashes.

4. High-sugar fruits: While fruits are generally a healthy choice, some are higher in sugar than others. High-sugar fruits to avoid or limit on a low blood sugar diet include bananas, grapes, and melons.

5. Alcohol: Alcohol can cause blood sugar levels to fluctuate and should be consumed in moderation or avoided altogether.

By avoiding or limiting these foods, individuals with hypoglycemia can help prevent blood sugar spikes and crashes and promote stable blood sugar levels throughout the day. It is important to work with a healthcare provider or registered dietitian to develop a personalized low blood sugar diet plan that meets individual nutritional needs and supports stable blood sugar levels.

Explanation of foods that can cause blood sugar spikes and crashes, such as refined carbohydrates and sugary drinks

Foods that are high in refined carbohydrates and added sugars can cause blood sugar levels to spike and then crash shortly thereafter. When we consume refined carbohydrates or sugary drinks, the body quickly breaks down the carbohydrates into glucose, which enters the bloodstream and causes a rapid increase in blood sugar levels.

In response, the pancreas releases insulin, a hormone that helps transport glucose into the body's cells for energy. However, when we consume large amounts of refined carbohydrates or added sugars, the body may produce too much insulin, causing blood sugar levels to drop rapidly. This can result in symptoms of hypoglycemia, such as dizziness, fatigue, and confusion. Refined carbohydrates include foods made with white flour, such as white bread, pasta, and pastries, as well as processed snacks and cereals. These foods are typically low in fiber and nutrients and are quickly broken down into glucose, causing a rapid increase in blood sugar levels. Sugary drinks, such as soda, fruit juice, and sports drinks, are high in added sugars and can cause blood sugar spikes. For example, a 12-ounce can of soda can contain up to 10 teaspoons of sugar, causing a rapid increase in blood sugar levels and a subsequent drop in blood sugar levels shortly thereafter.

By avoiding or limiting these foods, individuals with hypoglycemia can help prevent blood sugar spikes and crashes and promote stable blood sugar levels throughout the day. It is important to work with a healthcare provider or registered dietitian to develop a personalized low blood sugar diet plan that meets individual nutritional needs and supports stable blood sugar levels.

Overview of other lifestyle factors that can contribute to hypoglycemia, such as alcohol consumption and lack ofsleep

In addition to dietary factors, several lifestyle factors can contribute to hypoglycemia. Here are some examples:

1. Alcohol consumption: Alcohol can interfere with the liver's ability to release glucose into the bloodstream, which can cause blood sugar levels to drop rapidly. Additionally, alcohol can cause dehydration, which can also contribute to hypoglycemia.

2. Lack of sleep: A lack of sleep can cause hormonal imbalances, which can affect the body's ability to regulate blood sugar levels. Studies have shown that people who get less than 6 hours of sleep per night are more likely to experience blood sugar imbalances and hypoglycemia.

3. Stress: Stress can cause the body to release hormones such as cortisol, which can raise blood sugar levels in the short term. However, chronic stress can lead to

hormonal imbalances and contribute to hypoglycemia.

4. Medications: Certain medications, such as insulin and some types of oral diabetes medications, can cause hypoglycemia as a side effect.

5. Exercise: Regular exercise can help improve insulin sensitivity and promote stable blood sugar levels. However, strenuous exercise or exercise without proper fueling can cause blood sugar levels to drop rapidly.

By addressing these lifestyle factors, individuals with hypoglycemia can help manage their symptoms and promote stable blood sugar levels. It is important to work with a healthcare provider to identify any underlying causes of hypoglycemia and develop a comprehensive treatment plan that includes dietary and lifestyle modifications.

Meal Planning and Preparation On low blood sugar diet

Meal planning and preparation are essential components of a successful low blood sugar diet. Here are some tips for planning and preparing meals on a low blood sugar diet:

1. Plan ahead: Take time at the beginning of each week to plan out your meals and snacks for the week ahead. This can help ensure that you have a variety of healthy options on hand and can avoid last-minute, unhealthy food choices.

2. Use a food diary: Keeping a food diary can help you track your food intake and identify any patterns or triggers that may be contributing to your hypoglycemia.

3. Eat frequent, small meals: Eating small, frequent meals throughout the day can help maintain stable blood sugar levels. Aim to eat every 3-4 hours and include a balance of protein, complex carbohydrates, and healthy fats in each meal.

4. Choose whole foods: Focus on whole, nutrient-dense foods such as lean proteins, whole grains, fruits, and vegetables. These foods are generally lower in refined carbohydrates and added sugars and can help promote stable blood sugar levels.

5. Meal prep: Preparing meals and snacks in advance can help save time and ensure that you have healthy options on hand. Consider batch cooking and storing meals in the freezer for later use.

6. Use healthy cooking methods: Opt for healthy cooking methods such as baking,

grilling, and sautéing, rather than frying. This can help reduce the amount of added fats and calories in your meals.

By following these tips, individuals with hypoglycemia can create a balanced, nutritious, and delicious low blood sugar diet plan that supports stable blood sugar levels and promotes overall health and wellbeing.

Strategies for keeping bloos sugar level stable

Strategies for planning and preparing meals and snacks to keep blood sugar levels stable throughout the day

Planning and preparing meals and snacks can help individuals with hypoglycemia keep their blood sugar levels stable throughout the day. Here are some strategies for doing so:

1. Include protein in every meal and snack: Protein can help slow down the absorption of carbohydrates and prevent blood sugar spikes. Examples of high-protein foods include eggs, lean meats, poultry, fish, beans, and nuts.

2. Choose complex carbohydrates: Complex carbohydrates, such as whole grains, fruits, and vegetables, are digested more slowly than refined carbohydrates, such as white bread and sugary snacks. This slower digestion can help maintain stable blood sugar levels.

3. Avoid sugary drinks and snacks: Sugary drinks and snacks can cause rapid spikes and drops in blood sugar levels. Opt for water or unsweetened beverages and choose snacks that are low in sugar and high in protein and fiber.

4. Eat small, frequent meals: Eating small, frequent meals throughout the day can

help maintain stable blood sugar levels. Aim to eat every 3-4 hours and include a balance of protein, complex carbohydrates, and healthy fats in each meal.

5. Use healthy cooking methods: Opt for healthy cooking methods such as baking, grilling, and sautéing, rather than frying. This can help reduce the amount of added fats and calories in your meals.

6. Consider meal prep: Preparing meals and snacks in advance can help ensure that you have healthy options on hand and can avoid last-minute, unhealthy food choices. Consider batch cooking and storing meals in the freezer for later use.

By following these strategies, individuals with hypoglycemia can create a balanced, nutritious, and delicious low blood sugar diet plan that supports stable blood sugar levels and promotes overall health and wellbeing. It is important to work with a healthcare provider or registered dietitian to develop a personalized meal plan that meets your individual needs and preferences.

Tips for eating out and managing social situations while on a low blood sugar diet

Managing social situations and eating out can be challenging while on a low blood sugar diet. Here are some tips to help individuals with hypoglycemia navigate these situations:

1. Plan ahead: Research the restaurant or social event beforehand and look for menu options that fit within the principles of a low blood sugar diet. Many restaurants now have their menus

available online, which can help with planning ahead.

2. Ask questions: Don't be afraid to ask the server or host questions about how the food is prepared and what ingredients are used. This can help you make informed decisions about what to order.

3. Be mindful of portions: Restaurant portions are often much larger than what is recommended for a balanced meal. Consider asking for a smaller portion or splitting a meal with a friend.

4. Be prepared with snacks: If you are attending a social event where food options may be limited, consider bringing your own snacks, such as a protein bar or nuts, to help stabilize blood sugar levels.

5. Avoid sugary drinks: Opt for water or unsweetened beverages instead of sugary drinks, which can cause rapid spikes and drops in blood sugar levels.

6. Communicate with others: Let your friends or family know about your dietary needs and preferences so they can support you in making healthy choices while socializing.

Remember, it is important to enjoy social situations and not feel restricted by a low blood sugar diet. With some planning and preparation, individuals with hypoglycemia can continue to enjoy social events and dining out while still maintaining stable blood sugar levels.

Monitoring and Adjusting low blood sugar diet

Monitoring and adjusting a low blood sugar diet is an important aspect of managing hypoglycemia. Here are some tips for monitoring and adjusting the diet:

1. Monitor blood sugar levels: Regularly checking blood sugar levels can help individuals with hypoglycemia determine if their diet is working to maintain stable blood sugar levels. This can be done through finger-stick tests or continuous glucose monitoring.

2. Keep a food diary: Keeping a food diary can help individuals track what they are eating and how it affects their blood sugar levels. This can help identify patterns and make adjustments to the diet as needed.

3. Work with a healthcare provider or registered dietitian: Healthcare providers and registered dietitians can help individuals with hypoglycemia create a personalized meal plan and make adjustments to the diet as needed. They can also provide guidance on monitoring blood sugar levels and adjusting medications if necessary.

4. Adjust the diet based on individual needs: The principles of a low blood sugar diet are a guideline, but it is important to make adjustments based on individual needs and preferences. For example, some individuals may need to eat more frequent meals or include more protein in their diet.

5. Be patient: It may take some time to find the right balance of foods and meal timing that works to maintain stable blood sugar levels. Be patient and continue to monitor and adjust the diet as needed.

By monitoring and adjusting the diet as needed, individuals with hypoglycemia can create a sustainable and effective low blood sugar diet that supports stable blood sugar levels and overall health and wellbeing.

Importance of monitoring blood sugar levels and adjusting the diet as needed

Monitoring blood sugar levels and adjusting the diet as needed is crucial for managing hypoglycemia and maintaining stable blood sugar levels. By regularly checking blood sugar levels and keeping track of what foods are being eaten, individuals with hypoglycemia can identify patterns and make adjustments to their diet as necessary. For example, if someone notices that their blood sugar levels tend to drop too low after a certain meal, they can make adjustments to that meal, such as reducing the amount of carbohydrates or increasing the amount of protein. Similarly, if someone's blood sugar levels tend to spike after consuming certain foods, they can make adjustments to avoid those foods or consume them in smaller amounts. Working with a healthcare provider or registered dietitian can also be helpful in making adjustments to the diet. These professionals can provide personalized guidance on nutrition and meal planning, as well as help with monitoring blood sugar levels and adjusting medications if necessary.

By monitoring blood sugar levels and adjusting the diet as needed, individuals with hypoglycemia can effectively manage their condition and reduce the risk of complications associated with unstable blood sugar levels.

Overview of medications and other medical interventions for hypoglycemia

There are several medications and medical interventions that can be used to manage hypoglycemia, depending on the underlying cause and severity of the condition. Here are some examples:

1. Glucose tablets or gels: In mild cases of hypoglycemia, consuming glucose tablets or gels can quickly raise blood sugar levels and alleviate symptoms.

2. Glucagon injections: In more severe cases of hypoglycemia, glucagon injections may be used. Glucagon is a hormone that raises blood sugar levels by stimulating the liver to release stored glucose.

3. Oral medications: For individuals with diabetes who are at risk of hypoglycemia, adjusting the dosage or timing of oral diabetes medications can help prevent episodes of low blood sugar.

4. Insulin therapy: For individuals with diabetes, adjusting the dosage or timing of insulin injections or using different types of insulin can help prevent hypoglycemia.

5. Other medications: In some cases, medications used to treat other conditions, such as beta blockers or quinine, can cause hypoglycemia. Adjusting or discontinuing these medications may be necessary to manage the condition.

It is important to work with a healthcare provider to determine the appropriate medications and interventions for managing hypoglycemia. In some cases, lifestyle changes, such as following a low blood sugar diet or increasing physical activity, may also be recommended as part of the treatment plan.

The Optimal Low blood Sugar Diet Recipe

A low blood sugar diet aims to prevent spikes and crashes in blood sugar levels, which can cause symptoms such as fatigue, dizziness, and confusion. Here are three recipes for low blood sugar diet meals:

Scrambled Eggs with Vegetables

Ingredients:
* 2 large eggs
* 1/4 cup of chopped onion
* 1/4 cup of chopped red pepper
* 1/4 cup of chopped mushrooms
* 1 tablespoon of olive oil
* Salt and pepper to taste

Instructions:

1. Heat the olive oil in a non-stick skillet over medium heat.
2. Add the onion, red pepper, and mushrooms to the skillet and sauté for 3-4 minutes, until the vegetables are tender.
3. In a separate bowl, whisk the eggs with salt and pepper to taste.
4. Pour the eggs over the vegetables in the skillet and stir constantly until the eggs are cooked.
5. Serve hot.

Grilled Chicken Salad

Ingredients:
* 4 oz. of grilled chicken breast
* 2 cups of mixed salad greens
* 1/4 cup of cherry tomatoes
* 1/4 cup of sliced cucumber
* 1 tablespoon of olive oil
* 1 tablespoon of balsamic vinegar

* Salt and pepper to taste

Instructions:
1. Cut the grilled chicken breast into bite-sized pieces.
2. In a large bowl, mix together the salad greens, cherry tomatoes, and sliced cucumber.
3. Drizzle the olive oil and balsamic vinegar over the salad, and season with salt and pepper to taste.
4. Top the salad with the grilled chicken pieces.
5. Serve immediately.

Greek Yogurt Parfait

Ingredients:
* 1 cup of plain Greek yogurt
* 1/2 cup of mixed berries
* 1/4 cup of chopped walnuts

* 1 tablespoon of honey

Instructions:
1. In a small bowl, mix together the Greek yogurt and honey.
2. In a separate bowl, mix together the mixed berries and chopped walnuts.
3. Layer the Greek yogurt mixture and the berry mixture in a glass or bowl.
4. Serve chilled.

Low Carb Scrambled Eggs with Spinach and Feta Cheese

Ingredients:
* 3 eggs
* 1 cup spinach, chopped
* 1/4 cup feta cheese, crumbled
* 1 tablespoon butter
* Salt and pepper to taste

Instructions:
1. Beat the eggs in a bowl and add salt and pepper to taste.
2. Melt the butter in a non-stick pan over medium heat.
3. Add the chopped spinach and sauté for a few minutes until wilted.
4. Pour the beaten eggs into the pan and stir until they start to set.
5. Sprinkle the crumbled feta cheese over the eggs and continue stirring until the eggs are fully cooked.

Low Carb Chicken and Broccoli Stir Fry

Ingredients:
* 1 pound boneless skinless chicken breasts, cut into small pieces
* 2 cups broccoli florets
* 1 red bell pepper, sliced
* 1/4 cup soy sauce

* 2 tablespoons olive oil
* 1 tablespoon honey
* 1 tablespoon cornstarch
* 1 teaspoon minced garlic

1. Instructions:
2. In a small bowl, whisk together the soy sauce, honey, cornstarch, and minced garlic.
3. Heat the olive oil in a large skillet over medium-high heat.
4. Add the chicken to the skillet and sauté until browned on all sides.
5. Add the broccoli and red bell pepper to the skillet and stir-fry for a few minutes until tender-crisp.
6. Pour the soy sauce mixture over the chicken and vegetables and stir-fry for another minute or two until the sauce thickens and coats the chicken and vegetables.

Low Carb Greek Salad

Ingredients:
* 2 cups chopped romaine lettuce
* 1/2 cup chopped cucumber
* 1/2 cup cherry tomatoes, halved
* 1/4 cup crumbled feta cheese
* 2 tablespoons olive oil
* 1 tablespoon lemon juice
* 1/2 teaspoon dried oregano
* Salt and pepper to taste
1. Instructions:
2. In a large bowl, combine the chopped romaine lettuce, chopped cucumber, and halved cherry tomatoes.
3. In a small bowl, whisk together the olive oil, lemon juice, dried oregano, salt, and pepper.
4. Pour the dressing over the salad and toss to combine.

5. Sprinkle the crumbled feta cheese over the salad before serving.

Quinoa Salad

Ingredients:
* 1 cup quinoa, rinsed and drained
* 2 cups water
* 1/2 teaspoon salt
* 1/4 cup chopped fresh parsley
* 1/4 cup chopped fresh mint
* 1/4 cup chopped red onion
* 1/4 cup chopped walnuts
* 1/4 cup dried cranberries
* 1/4 cup crumbled feta cheese
* 2 tablespoons olive oil
* 2 tablespoons fresh lemon juice
* 1 clove garlic, minced

Instructions:

1. In a medium saucepan, combine quinoa, water, and salt. Bring to a boil over high heat. Reduce heat to low and simmer for 15-20 minutes, or until quinoa is tender and water is absorbed.

2. In a large bowl, combine cooked quinoa, parsley, mint, red onion, walnuts, cranberries, and feta cheese.

3. In a small bowl, whisk together olive oil, lemon juice, and garlic. Pour over quinoa mixture and toss to coat.

4. Serve at room temperature or chilled.

Baked Sweet Potato Fries

Ingredients:
* 2 medium sweet potatoes, peeled and cut into fries
* 2 tablespoons olive oil
* 1 teaspoon paprika
* 1/2 teaspoon garlic powder

* 1/2 teaspoon salt
* 1/4 teaspoon black pepper

Instructions:
1. Preheat oven to 425°F.
2. In a large bowl, combine sweet potato fries, olive oil, paprika, garlic powder, salt, and black pepper. Toss to coat.
3. Spread sweet potato fries in a single layer on a baking sheet lined with parchment paper.
4. Bake for 25-30 minutes, or until fries are crispy and tender.
5. Serve hot.

Turkey and Vegetable Stir Fry

Ingredients:
* 1 pound turkey breast, cut into thin strips
* 1 tablespoon cornstarch

* 1 tablespoon soy sauce
* 1 tablespoon sesame oil
* 1/4 teaspoon black pepper
* 1 tablespoon olive oil
* 1 red bell pepper, sliced
* 1 yellow bell pepper, sliced
* 1 medium zucchini, sliced
* 1 medium carrot, sliced
* 2 cloves garlic, minced
* 1/4 cup chicken broth

Instructions:
1. In a medium bowl, combine turkey breast, cornstarch, soy sauce, sesame oil, and black pepper. Toss to coat.
2. Heat olive oil in a large skillet over medium-high heat. Add turkey breast and cook for 3-4 minutes, or until browned on all sides.

3. Add bell peppers, zucchini, carrot, and garlic to the skillet. Cook for 5-7 minutes, or until vegetables are tender.

4. Add chicken broth to the skillet and stir to combine. Cook for an additional 2-3 minutes, or until sauce thickens.

5. Serve hot.

Omelet with Vegetables

Ingredients:
* 2 large eggs
* 1 tablespoon olive oil
* 1/2 cup chopped vegetables (such as bell peppers, onions, and spinach)
* Salt and pepper to taste

Instructions:
1. Heat olive oil in a nonstick pan over medium heat.

2. Add the vegetables and cook until they are tender, about 5 minutes.
3. Beat the eggs in a bowl and add salt and pepper to taste.
4. Pour the egg mixture into the pan and cook until set, about 3-4 minutes.
5. Fold the omelet in half and serve.

Chicken and Vegetable Stir Fry

Ingredients:
* 1 pound boneless, skinless chicken breast, sliced into strips
* 2 tablespoons vegetable oil
* 1 cup sliced vegetables (such as broccoli, bell peppers, and carrots)
* 1/4 cup low-sugar teriyaki sauce
* Salt and pepper to taste

Instructions:

1. Heat the vegetable oil in a large pan or wok over high heat.
2. Add the chicken and cook until browned on all sides, about 5 minutes.
3. Add the vegetables and stir fry until they are tender, about 3-4 minutes.
4. Add the teriyaki sauce and cook until the chicken and vegetables are coated, about 1-2 minutes.
5. Season with salt and pepper to taste and serve.

Greek Yogurt with Berries

Ingredients:
* 1 cup plain Greek yogurt
* 1/2 cup mixed berries (such as strawberries, blueberries, and raspberries)
* 1 tablespoon honey

Instructions:

1. In a bowl, mix together the Greek yogurt and honey.
2. Top with the mixed berries and serve.

Roasted Sweet Potato Fries

Ingredients:
* 2 large sweet potatoes, peeled and sliced into wedges
* 2 tablespoons olive oil
* 1 teaspoon garlic powder
* 1 teaspoon paprika
* Salt and pepper to taste

Instructions:
1. Preheat the oven to 400°F (200°C).
2. In a bowl, mix together the olive oil, garlic powder, paprika, salt, and pepper.
3. Add the sweet potato wedges and toss to coat.

4. Spread the sweet potato wedges on a baking sheet in a single layer.
5. Roast for 20-25 minutes, flipping halfway through, until the sweet potato fries are tender and crispy.
6. Serve hot.

Vegetable Omelette

Ingredients:
* 2 eggs
* 1/4 cup diced onions
* 1/4 cup diced bell peppers
* 1/4 cup diced mushrooms
* Salt and pepper to taste
* 1 tbsp olive oil

Instructions:
1. Beat the eggs in a bowl and add salt and pepper.

2. Heat the olive oil in a non-stick pan over medium heat.

3. Add the onions, bell peppers, and mushrooms to the pan and sauté for 2-3 minutes.

4. Pour the egg mixture into the pan and cook for 2-3 minutes or until the edges start to set.

5. Flip the omelette over and cook for another 1-2 minutes or until fully cooked.

6. Serve hot.

Chicken and Broccoli Stir Fry

Ingredients:
* 1 boneless, skinless chicken breast, sliced
* 2 cups broccoli florets
* 1/4 cup sliced onions
* 1/4 cup sliced bell peppers
* 1 tbsp olive oil

* Salt and pepper to taste

Instructions:
1. Heat the olive oil in a pan over medium-high heat.
2. Add the sliced chicken to the pan and cook for 5-7 minutes or until fully cooked.
3. Add the broccoli, onions, and bell peppers to the pan and sauté for 2-3 minutes.
4. Season with salt and pepper to taste.
5. Serve hot.

Greek Yogurt Parfait.

Ingredients:
* 1/2 cup plain Greek yogurt
* 1/4 cup chopped mixed nuts
* 1/4 cup mixed berries
* 1 tbsp honey

Instructions:
1. In a small bowl, layer the Greek yogurt, chopped nuts, and mixed berries.
2. Drizzle honey over the top.
3. Serve chilled.

Turkey Lettuce Wraps

Ingredients:
* 1 lb ground turkey
* 1/4 cup diced onions
* 1/4 cup diced bell peppers
* 1/4 cup diced mushrooms
* 1 tbsp olive oil
* Salt and pepper to taste
* Lettuce leaves for wrapping

Instructions:
1. Heat the olive oil in a pan over medium-high heat.

2. Add the diced onions, bell peppers, and mushrooms to the pan and sauté for 2-3 minutes.
3. Add the ground turkey to the pan and cook for 5-7 minutes or until fully cooked.
4. Season with salt and pepper to taste.
5. Spoon the turkey mixture onto lettuce leaves and wrap.
6. Serve immediately.

Greek Yogurt with Berries and Nuts

Ingredients:
* 1 cup plain Greek yogurt
* 1/2 cup mixed berries (such as blueberries, raspberries, and strawberries)
* 1/4 cup chopped nuts (such as almonds, walnuts, or pecans)

Instructions:
1. Place the Greek yogurt in a bowl.

2. Top with the mixed berries and chopped nuts.

3. Enjoy as a snack or breakfast.

Egg and Veggie Breakfast Wrap

Ingredients:
* 1 whole-wheat wrap
* 2 eggs, scrambled
* 1/4 cup chopped vegetables (such as bell peppers, onions, and mushrooms)
* 1 tablespoon olive oil

Instructions:
1. Heat the olive oil in a pan over medium heat.
2. Add the chopped vegetables and sauté until softened.
3. Add the scrambled eggs and cook until firm.

4. Place the egg and veggie mixture onto the whole-wheat wrap.
5. Roll up the wrap and enjoy as a breakfast or lunch option.

Quinoa and Vegetable Stir-Fry

Ingredients:
* 1 cup cooked quinoa
* 1/2 cup chopped vegetables (such as broccoli, bell peppers, and onions)
* 1 tablespoon olive oil
* 1 tablespoon low-sodium soy sauce

Instructions:
1. Heat the olive oil in a pan over medium heat.
2. Add the chopped vegetables and sauté until softened.
3. Add the cooked quinoa and low-sodium soy sauce to the pan.

4. Stir until all ingredients are combined and heated through.
5. Serve as a side dish or main course.

Grilled Chicken and Vegetable Skewers

Ingredients:
* 1 pound boneless, skinless chicken breast, cut into cubes
* 1 cup chopped vegetables (such as bell peppers, onions, and zucchini)
* 2 tablespoons olive oil
* 1 teaspoon dried herbs (such as oregano or thyme)

Instructions:
1. Preheat a grill or grill pan to medium-high heat.
2. Thread the chicken cubes and chopped vegetables onto skewers.

3. Brush the skewers with olive oil and sprinkle with dried herbs.

4. Grill the skewers for 10-12 minutes, turning occasionally, until the chicken is cooked through.

5. Serve as a main course with a side salad or cooked grains.

Turkey and Hummus Lettuce Wraps

Ingredients:
* 4 large lettuce leaves
* 4 slices of deli turkey
* 4 tablespoons hummus
* 1/4 cup chopped vegetables (such as bell peppers, onions, and carrots)

Instructions:
1. Lay out the lettuce leaves and place a slice of deli turkey on each.

2. Spread 1 tablespoon of hummus on top of the turkey.
3. Top with chopped vegetables.
4. Roll up the lettuce leaves and enjoy as a lunch or snack option.

Turkey and Veggie Wrap:

Ingredients:
* 1 large whole-wheat tortilla wrap
* 3 oz sliced turkey breast
* 1/4 avocado, sliced
* 1/4 cup shredded carrots
* 1/4 cup baby spinach leaves
* 1/4 cup cherry tomatoes, halved
* 1 tablespoon hummus

Instructions:
1. Lay the tortilla wrap flat and spread the hummus evenly over the surface.

2. Add the turkey breast, avocado, shredded carrots, spinach leaves, and cherry tomatoes.
3. Roll the wrap tightly, tucking in the ends as you go.
4. Cut the wrap in half and enjoy!

Quinoa Salad:

Ingredients:
* 1 cup cooked quinoa
* 1/2 cup cooked black beans
* 1/2 cup chopped bell pepper
* 1/2 cup chopped cucumber
* 1/4 cup chopped red onion
* 1/4 cup chopped cilantro
* 2 tablespoons olive oil
* 2 tablespoons lime juice
* Salt and pepper to taste

Instructions:

1. In a large bowl, combine the cooked quinoa, black beans, bell pepper, cucumber, red onion, and cilantro.

2. In a separate small bowl, whisk together the olive oil, lime juice, salt, and pepper.

3. Pour the dressing over the salad and toss to combine.

4. Serve chilled or at room temperature.

Egg and Veggie Scramble:

Ingredients:
* 2 eggs
* 1/4 cup chopped bell pepper
* 1/4 cup chopped onion
* 1/4 cup chopped mushroom
* 1 tablespoon olive oil
* Salt and pepper to taste

Instructions:

1. In a small bowl, whisk together the eggs with a pinch of salt and pepper.
2. Heat the olive oil in a nonstick skillet over medium heat.
3. Add the bell pepper, onion, and mushroom and sauté for a few minutes until the vegetables are tender.
4. Pour the eggs into the skillet and stir continuously until the eggs are cooked through.
5. Serve hot and enjoy!

Quinoa Bowl with Vegetables and Chicken

Ingredients:
* 1 cup of quinoa
* 1 chicken breast, sliced
* 1 cup of broccoli, chopped
* 1 cup of carrots, chopped
* 1 tbsp olive oil
* Salt and pepper to taste

Instructions:
1. Cook quinoa according to package instructions.
2. Heat olive oil in a pan over medium heat.
3. Add chicken and cook until golden brown, about 5 minutes.
4. Add vegetables and cook until tender, about 5-7 minutes.
5. Season with salt and pepper.
6. Serve vegetables and chicken on top of the cooked quinoa.

Greek Yogurt Parfait

Ingredients:
* 1 cup of plain Greek yogurt
* 1/2 cup of mixed berries
* 1/4 cup of granola
* 1 tbsp honey

Instructions:
1. Mix Greek yogurt with honey in a bowl.
2. Layer yogurt mixture, berries, and granola in a glass.
3. Serve immediately.

Chickpea and Spinach Salad

Ingredients:
* 1 can of chickpeas, drained and rinsed
* 2 cups of spinach leaves
* 1/4 cup of sliced almonds
* 1/4 cup of crumbled feta cheese
* 2 tbsp olive oil
* 1 tbsp lemon juice
* Salt and pepper to taste

Instructions:
1. In a large bowl, mix chickpeas, spinach, almonds, and feta cheese.

2. In a small bowl, whisk olive oil and lemon juice together.

3. Pour dressing over salad and toss to combine.

4. Season with salt and pepper.

5. Serve immediately.

Turkey and Vegetable Stir Fry

Ingredients:
* 1 lb of ground turkey
* 1 cup of broccoli florets
* 1 cup of snow peas
* 1 cup of carrots, sliced
* 1/4 cup of soy sauce
* 2 tbsp olive oil
* Salt and pepper to taste

Instructions:
1. Heat olive oil in a pan over medium heat.

2. Add ground turkey and cook until browned, about 5-7 minutes.

3. Add vegetables and cook until tender, about 5-7 minutes.

4. Add soy sauce and stir to combine.

5. Season with salt and pepper.

6. Serve immediately.

Egg and Veggie Scramble

Ingredients:
* 2 large eggs
* 1/4 cup chopped onions
* 1/4 cup chopped bell peppers
* 1/4 cup chopped mushrooms
* 1 tablespoon olive oil
* Salt and pepper to taste

Instructions:
1. Heat the olive oil in a non-stick pan over medium heat.

2. Add the onions, bell peppers, and mushrooms and sauté for 2-3 minutes, until the vegetables are tender.

3. Beat the eggs in a bowl and season with salt and pepper.

4. Pour the eggs into the pan with the vegetables and scramble until the eggs are cooked through.

5. Serve hot.

Grilled Chicken and Vegetable Skewers

Ingredients:
* 2 boneless, skinless chicken breasts
* 1 zucchini, sliced
* 1 red bell pepper, chopped
* 1 yellow bell pepper, chopped
* 1/4 cup olive oil
* 1/4 cup balsamic vinegar
* 1 tablespoon Dijon mustard
* Salt and pepper to taste

Instructions:
1. Preheat a grill or grill pan to medium-high heat.
2. Cut the chicken into bite-sized pieces and thread onto skewers along with the sliced zucchini and chopped bell peppers.
3. In a small bowl, whisk together the olive oil, balsamic vinegar, Dijon mustard, salt, and pepper.
4. Brush the chicken and vegetables with the marinade.
5. Grill the skewers for 8-10 minutes, turning occasionally, until the chicken is cooked through.
6. Serve hot.

Cauliflower Rice Stir-Fry

Ingredients:
* 1 head cauliflower, grated or chopped into small pieces

* 1/2 cup chopped onions
* 1/2 cup chopped carrots
* 1/2 cup chopped broccoli
* 1/4 cup soy sauce
* 1 tablespoon sesame oil
* 1 tablespoon olive oil
* Salt and pepper to taste

Instructions:
1. Heat the olive oil and sesame oil in a large pan over medium heat.
2. Add the onions, carrots, and broccoli and sauté for 2-3 minutes, until the vegetables are tender.
3. Add the cauliflower and stir-fry for another 3-4 minutes, until the cauliflower is tender but still slightly crunchy.
4. Add the soy sauce and stir-fry for an additional 1-2 minutes, until the vegetables are coated with the sauce.
5. Season with salt and pepper to taste.

6. Serve hot.

Oatmeal and Blueberry Breakfast Bars

Ingredients:
* 2 cups old-fashioned rolled oats
* 1 cup whole wheat flour
* 1 tsp baking powder
* 1 tsp ground cinnamon
* 1/4 tsp salt
* 1/2 cup unsweetened applesauce
* 1/4 cup honey
* 1/4 cup unsweetened almond milk
* 2 tbsp coconut oil, melted
* 1 egg
* 1 cup blueberries

Instructions:
1. Preheat the oven to 350°F and line a 9x9-inch baking pan with parchment paper.

2. In a large bowl, mix together the oats, flour, baking powder, cinnamon, and salt.

3. In a separate bowl, whisk together the applesauce, honey, almond milk, coconut oil, and egg until well combined.

4. Pour the wet ingredients into the dry ingredients and stir until just combined.

5. Gently fold in the blueberries.

6. Pour the batter into the prepared pan and smooth out the top.

7. Bake for 25-30 minutes or until a toothpick inserted in the center comes out clean.

8. Let the bars cool in the pan for 10 minutes before slicing and serving.

Turkey and Sweet Potato Skillet

Ingredients:
* 1 lb ground turkey
* 1 tbsp olive oil
* 1 onion, chopped

* 2 garlic cloves, minced
* 1 sweet potato, peeled and diced
* 1 red bell pepper, chopped
* 1 tsp ground cumin
* 1 tsp paprika
* 1/4 tsp salt
* 1/4 tsp black pepper
* 1 can (14.5 oz) diced tomatoes
* 1/4 cup chopped fresh cilantro

Instructions:
1. Heat the olive oil in a large skillet over medium heat.
2. Add the ground turkey and cook, breaking it up with a wooden spoon, until browned and cooked through, about 8 minutes.
3. Add the onion, garlic, sweet potato, and red bell pepper to the skillet and cook until the vegetables are softened, about 5 minutes.

4. Add the cumin, paprika, salt, and black pepper to the skillet and stir to combine.
5. Pour in the diced tomatoes and stir to combine.
6. Reduce the heat to low and let the skillet simmer until the sweet potato is tender and the flavors have melded, about 10-15 minutes.
7. Stir in the chopped cilantro and serve.

Lemon Garlic Shrimp and Broccoli

Ingredients:
* 1 lb raw shrimp, peeled and deveined
* 2 tbsp olive oil
* 2 garlic cloves, minced
* 1 lemon, zested and juiced
* 1/4 tsp salt
* 1/4 tsp black pepper
* 4 cups broccoli florets

Instructions:
1. Heat the olive oil in a large skillet over medium-high heat.
2. Add the shrimp and cook until pink and cooked through, about 3-4 minutes per side.
3. Add the garlic to the skillet and cook for 30 seconds or until fragrant.
4. Add the lemon zest, lemon juice, salt, and black pepper to the skillet and stir to combine.
5. Add the broccoli to the skillet and stir to coat in the sauce.
6. Cover the skillet and let the broccoli steam for 5-7 minutes or until tender.
7. Serve the shrimp and broccoli

CONCLUSION

In conclusion, a low blood sugar diet can be an effective way to manage hypoglycemia and maintain stable blood sugar levels throughout the day. The key principles of a low blood sugar diet include eating small, frequent meals that are balanced in macronutrients and avoiding refined carbohydrates and added sugars. Lean proteins, whole grains, vegetables, and healthy fats are all good choices for those following a low blood sugar diet. Meal planning and preparation are important strategies for keeping blood sugar levels stable throughout the day, and there are also tips for managing social situations and eating out while following a low blood sugar diet. Monitoring blood sugar levels and adjusting the diet as needed, with the guidance of a healthcare provider or registered dietitian, is crucial for effectively managing hypoglycemia.

In addition to dietary changes, there are also medications and medical interventions that can be used to manage hypoglycemia. By taking a comprehensive approach to managing the condition, individuals with hypoglycemia can reduce the risk of complications and lead a healthy, active lifestyle.

Printed in Great Britain
by Amazon

22588605R00050